Marketing for the Holistic Practitioner

Build a Thriving Holistic Health Care Practice.

A Simple Low Cost Guide For
Therapists and Practitioners
on Getting and Keeping Your Clients.

Build a Thriving Holistic Health Care Practice
A Simple Low Cost Guide For Therapists
and Practitioners on Getting and Keeping Your Clients
by Michelle A. Vandepas

Published by Conscious Destiny Productions, Inc.

© December, 2003 Michelle A. Vandepas

The legal fine print:

~~~~

In other words, read and enjoy this book. Use the parts that inspire and motivate you, ignore the rest. Use your own common sense and intuition when deciding. Please don't hold me responsible for your failures, and I won't take credit for your successes. Most of all, have fun and enjoy your precious time on earth. Michelle

*A*cknowledgments

Thank you to the Rock Creek Canyon Art Group who has kept me motivated, inspired and who helped with the early stages of my manuscript: DeAnne Dingwall, Susan Blue, Kathryn Wallace and Barbara Blake.

Also many thanks to the Accountability Group of Montague's for your continuing support, especially Wendy for her email encouragements and 'get off your butt' directives.

Thanks to my good friend Susan Tinkle for help in editing this project and for her years of friendship and encouragement.

And of course to my husband of over 22 years, Thanks Bob.

"Often people attempt to live their lives backwards. They try to have more things or more money to do more of what they want, so they will be happier. The way it actually works is in reverse. You must first be who you really are, then do what you need to do to have what you want." Margaret Young

"I am already kindly disposed towards you. My friendship it is not in my power to give: this is a gift which no man can make, it is not in our own power: a sound and healthy friendship is the growth of time and circumstance, it will spring up and thrive." William Wordsworth

"Every business is built on friendship." J. C. Penney

Table of Contents

*I*ntroduction

"It is not the goal to get out of here alive, but to heal ourselves." Dr. Spencer Woolley

Welcome to "Marketing for the Holistic Practitioner- A simple low cost marketing guide for therapists and practitioners." After reading this book and working with the exercises, it is my hope that you join the many holistic practitioners who are working at their passion of healing and thriving.

Over the past ten years I have met hundreds of holistic practitioners. Some were struggling financially and others were supporting themselves and providing a comfortable living for their families. As a consultant, I am often asked what makes one practitioner financially successful while another scrapes by week to week. What are the skills needed to build a practice? My answer? It is partially a combination of *being and doing.*

Being" the best person and practitioner, you can be, and doing the work it takes to be successful.

Basic marketing principles when followed, can help you live your dreams, follow your passions, and make a viable, secure living while doing so!

The holistic industry has a special place in my heart. In 1987 I was diagnosed with Chronic Fatigue Syndrome along with Epstein Barr and Mononucleosis. Somehow I managed to keep my computer business running with a myriad of symptoms that included migraine headaches, permanently swollen lymph glands, arthritis, and extreme tiredness. Put simply, my body was worn out, burned out, and I was depleted, emotionally and spiritually.

My health journey had not yet taken me into the holistic world. And then a friend introduced me to Dr. Spencer Woolley, a homeopathic physician. The first conversation I had with him was foreign to me, and included strange notions such as a nutritious healing diet. However, I connected to him and his message. More importantly, I trusted him and I trusted the modality. I started to feel hope that someday I would be well again.

Dr. Spencer imparted a calm center; he was grounded, patient, and knowledgeable. He helped me see past my sickness to a world of wellness. This was a world to which I desperately wanted to belong, and so I began my long journey back to health. Along the way Dr. Spencer introduced me to other wonderful practitioners, and many other types of therapies. Slowly I began to learn and study, and I recovered my physical health and my emotional well-being.

My studies and therapies included massage, chiropractic and acupuncture as well as more controversial therapies such as energy work, chakra balancing and soul retrieval. All the modalities fascinated me, - there was so much to learn! I worked with many holistic practitioners who cared about guiding me through my personal journey, not just my treatment.

Almost everyone I encountered in the holistic world gave me time and space to discover who I was and which tools and therapies I should use. This world was different from the medical regimens I was used to. These therapists were supportive, encouraging and nonjudgmental.

After regaining my health, I wanted to use all this new knowledge to help others. So, with two partners, (one of whom was Spencer Woolley the wonderful homeopath who had started me on my journey), I founded a holistic company manufacturing homeopathic remedies and a testing device to work with the remedies and patients. We sold our products to alternative clinics and practitioners and we did quite well.

I soon discovered that many practitioners didn't know how to market themselves much less build a practice, so I used my business and marketing background to train our new customers.

Over the next seven years I trained hundreds of clinicians who came from different spiritual and religious beliefs and practiced all types of therapies. I've worked with homeopaths, massage therapists, nutritionists, born-again Christians and pagans.

However, I found a common thread binding each practitioner. It was (and is) a deep understanding that healing comes from within, using forces not always seen. Healing builds upon a foundation based upon spiritual laws.

I loved working with these healers.

All the therapists were immensely gifted at their craft. However, many of them presumed that if you put an ad in the yellow pages, people would come knocking. Others thought that writing one article in the community newspaper, or giving away free services for a month would build their practice into a thriving business. I wish it were so, but it's simply not enough.

Marketing this industry has its own set of challenges: the public is uneducated, some modalities are not yet scientifically proven according to a Western medical model; often the training of therapists is unregulated. The public is skeptical. New clients get confused with all the options available. They discover there is a new way to approach health that defies the notion of a quick fix cure that our society is used to. They are overwhelmed with new information and often believe that they don't have time or money to follow up with a holistic plan.

In the past, prospective clients often found a lack of professionalism within the industry. Some practitioners worked from their living room, or perhaps they wore jeans and a t-shirt without thought for their presentation as a professional. The clients didn't return, and, not knowing how to really find a new practitioner, gave up altogether.

The therapists couldn't help this cycle. They didn't know how. Many had almost no business or marketing background. They struggled to learn how to market, how to present themselves, how to run their business and become successful.

After working with these therapists over many years, I have found there are only a few basic marketing guidelines that, when followed, helped their practices grow and thrive.

This book combines these marketing ideas, along with some observations, of what makes a successful practitioner. Perhaps you have picked up this book because you could use some new ideas. Maybe you are just curious. Either way, I hope you will find something new to spark your interest, or keep you motivated.

As a holistic health care practitioner, you are on the forefront of the future of healthcare. I applaud you. You are living your passion, and through this passion, guiding yourself and others to healing. You are working toward global wellness and healing of the planet.

I want you to be financially successful so that you may continue to do your work. If you learn how to make the business of healing indeed a *business*, then you may progress on your path and support yourself and your family financially.

I feel immense gratitude to all the health care practitioners and light workers who have helped me regain my health. Today my health is considered normal although, like everyone, I occasionally struggle with diet and exercise.

My healing continues, through a creative journey that combines holistic living, spiritual study and acceptance of self. This path has given me a gift of spiritual and creative strength and many lifelong friends. I thank them all.

My hope is that this book gives you some guidance in building your business so that you will also guide others on their journey toward wellness.

I'd love to hear your personal stories.

You can write to me at:

Conscious Destiny Productions, Inc.
1120 Rock Creek Canyon Road
Colorado Springs CO 80926

www.consciousdesitny.com
michelle@consciousdestiny.com

May each of you help heal the world, one person at a time.

Namaste

Michelle

The Exercises

"Words are a form of action, capable of influencing change." Ingrid Bengis

Throughout the book you will find some questions, and written exercises for you to complete. Please take the time to get out your favorite pen and paper to write down your thoughts as you are reading. These exercises are designed to tap your innermost feelings and thoughts about starting a business and promoting and marketing yourself. Using paper and pen will get your body involved in this process and help you get in touch with these feelings. When you come to a question, don't think too much, just write and allow your knowingness, your intuition, to guide your answers. Trust your first instinct and go with whatever feelings or thoughts you may have.

Keep in mind there are no right or wrong answers. These are exploratory exercises for you. It won't matter if you put down a silly answer or write something that doesn't seem relevant. Just answer the questions, as honestly as you can. After some soul-searching, you may choose to expand upon your answers. And after thinking for a day or a week about some of the chapters, you may find, you want to go back and write again.

Allow the process to evolve. Keep all of your writing, but don't share it with anyone else. This is for you and it is private, intimate, and safe.

You may find a specific ritual will help you stay focused and relaxed. Choose a time of day when you are least likely to be interrupted, so you can read and write in peace. If you have an office, sit at your desk, so that your subconscious mind kicks into work mode and helps to keep you focused. If you choose light a candle, say a prayer, meditate and give yourself permission to be successful at the process and in your practice. You may have feelings of fear, anxiety or uncertainty that come up in your body. Acknowledge these feelings, (take some Rescue Remedy if necessary!) and continue the work.

If you get stumped, try writing with your non dominant hand. This will help you connect with your heart more quickly, and force you to slow down as you write. The answers that come may surprise you!

This process of slowing down allows your thoughts to surface completely before you start to write. Then, as you write, your mind continues to process the thought until there is nothing left to say. Slowly, the next thought organically emerges for contemplation.

Whether you choose to write fast, write slow, on the computer, with pen or pencil or just think about your practice, the most important step is the self-reflection. Take the time to think about your journey and how to facilitate it.

Many of us are used to writing or typing so quickly that we condense our thoughts in the process of getting them down, and then we lose the full complexity of what we are trying to say.

So, here we go! Hang on for the ride, and most of all, embrace the process and have fun.

Commitment

"Commitment leads to action. Action brings your dream closer." Marcia Wieder

Now, I'm not going to kid you. Having a practice means that you have a business, and having a business means doing the planning, accounting, and marketing to keep it all running. This takes time, effort and energy, and most of all, commitment. You will be perfecting your craft, finding clients, making calls, writing letters, washing toilets. You will be doing it all when you manage your own business. As they say, the buck stops here.

Is owning your own business part of your dream? If not, stop here. Don't read any more of this book, or print any business cards. There are plenty of opportunities out there for good therapists; you can always go to work for someone else. Try working in a spa, holistic health center or health food store. Find another professional in a similar therapy you could work for.

If the idea of owning your own business is exciting to you, if you see possibilities and opportunity, rather than hard work and frustration, then *start now.*

Go past the fear, past the doubt and ignore your external and internal skeptic. Believe that you can find a way to make this dream come true. Yes it will be scary at times, but that's not a good reason to quit. You have to feel the fear and do it anyway.

Now for the good news. When you are doing all of this work for yourself, it doesn't seem as hard. In fact it can even be fun. Having your own business is full of rewards. You decide, plan and execute your fate. You are in charge. You can have a higher level of job satisfaction and the potential of a higher income. You can be creative and independent. But no more excuses! No more whining. As you know, the buck stops here!

Take a moment and create your ideal job.

- What does it look life?
- Are you working for someone else or for yourself?
- Where do you get the most job satisfaction?

So, will you commit? Are you ready to commit to yourself?

Will you treat your practice as a business or hobby? You can have a part-time business, or a full-time hobby, but only one of these will support you and your family financially. Which do you want for yourself?

If you are looking to build a thriving business, (either full or part-time) you will need to examine your thought processes. Do your subconscious thoughts support your commitment?

Is there a part of you that doubts your own ability?

Do you secretly think that you aren't worthy enough, experienced enough, or don't have enough schooling? Then that will be the outward impression you will give to others. They may think that you are still learning your craft and are not yet ready to open your business.

Perhaps you mistakenly give the impression that you are looking to practice on clients. You come across as unsure of your pricing, abilities and schedule. Clients think you are asking them to be your guinea pig. Put yourself in their place. Are you the type of therapist you would trust your own health and well being to?

If you introduce yourself with assurance, in a well thought out ten-second mini presentation, your future clients instantly connect with you as someone who is worthy of their trust. Your presentation, how you dress, and your level of confidence, will tell the world, and the universe, that you have committed. You will tell your clients that you have a serious business and that you are not just practicing a hobby.

Finish these sentences:

▸   When I meet someone new I come across to them as:

▸   I feel sure of my abilities when:

▸   I am unsure of my abilities when:

▸   I treat my business as a hobby when I:

Now, think back. Everything in your life that has been the most rewarding has required a major commitment from you. Not just the mental commitment, but also the physical commitment of *doing* every day. All your major accomplishments; raising your children, your swimming trophy from eighth grade, the beautiful garden that is in full bloom in August, becoming a certified therapist.

Before each of these accomplishments, there first came a commitment - a commitment that required follow through with action each day. After the commitment, then you gave personal attention, time, thought and preparation. It was all in the doing.

This action is a manifestation of your commitment. Once you commit, you must do, and it's this doing that adds up to results. You achieve your goals. Commitment comes from a place deep inside where you decide, and then every day re-affirm your decision.

Perhaps one day in the middle of the summer you find yourself sitting around at home lying on the couch watching Oprah and eating chocolate cookies. Now, of course we all need vacations, rest days, and times when we just goof off. But what if you are finding that you are on vacation day after day after day? Will this get you closer to your passions? This is a day to reaffirm your goals to yourself. Don't you want to look back on your life and be proud of what you have accomplished?

Most of us know what we need to do to get more clients, (and if you don't know, I'm going to tell you), but we are lazy by nature. Well, if not exactly lazy, we want the easiest way out. Artists always say, "If I had an agent, then I could just paint all day and let someone else sell for me." Nevertheless, we have to pay our dues, put brush to paint, or pen to paper, call a gallery, or, perhaps in your case, give a free mini massage. We have to believe in ourselves and get to work.

I presume that you have lots of ideas in your head to start your own business. You might even write down these ideas and tell all your friends, but now you just have to stop the procrastination and get out there and tell people what you do and follow through on your ideas.

At some point, you just have to take all the stuff you know in your head, and in the best Nike fashion, *Just Do It*. I promise you that having this approach to life will be the most important thing you can do for yourself. As I said, feel the fear, but do it anyway.

This book is going to help you. It will get you going, get you off your duff and give you some easy exercises to keep you focused. However, reading the book won't be enough. You'll have more ideas, but you still *gotta* do the work.

Sorry, but it's that simple. Now, it's time for you to commit. Are you ready? Will you do it? Are you ready to commit to yourself?

Commit to yourself, the universe and everything.

Do it now. . . and then, renew this commitment in your heart everyday.

▸ Write a paragraph now about what success looks like.

▸ How many clients do you have?

▸ What type of practice have you built?

▸ What do your clients look like?

Brainstorm the ideas and allow your inner mind to start committing.

Time Management

"Anything that is wasted effort represents wasted time. The best management of our time thus becomes linked inseparably with the best utilization of our efforts."
Ted W. Engstrom

Now that you have made a strong commitment to yourself, lets start analyzing how you spend your time each day. Does the time spent each day reflect your commitment?

The key to having a balanced life when starting a business is to make time - time for self nourishment, relaxation, play, friends, family and spirituality. However you will have to schedule the activities so that your interruptions can be minimized.

My consultant friend Mary decided to refocus her energy into building her business. However she had a girlfriend who called several times a day just to talk. They had talked often together for over a year, catching up, gossiping and supporting each other through life. But now, Mary was using her days to market herself, and the calls were getting distracting, taking away from her scheduled tasks. Mary tried using her Caller Id to screen calls and even tried just not answering the phone, but she found her friend would just hang up and keep calling until Mary would answer the phone. After a couple of weeks, their relationship got very tense. Finally, one day when Mary answered the phone, she just blew. "Don't you know I'm trying to work? How can you keep interrupting me when I am so far behind?" Her friend was aghast, she'd had no idea she was upsetting Mary by continuing to do what she had done for a whole year. Finally Mary had to come clean about her feelings, having to work during the day and schedule time to market her business. "I've committed to building my practice and I just don't have the free time I used to." She said, "Perhaps we can arrange to talk every Sunday after dinner."

Obviously you can see it would have been better had Mary been clear about her commitments and new responsibilities up front, before it came to a boiling point. However, as soon as she spoke her truth in a loving manner, her friend was supportive and even offered to help her distribute fliers to neighboring businesses.

What about you? Do you have any time leeches - people or things that take time away from your responsibilities? If so, it is *your* responsibility to speak up, tell others your plans, and schedule accordingly.

Maybe your problem just seems to be a lack of time. You have children, family, errands to run, and there just doesn't seem to be enough time in the day. Again, the skills you need are the same. Stay focused, schedule and prioritize. Focus on the important, and any urgency will take care of itself. You will find you have fewer emergencies coming up when you take a few moments to rank your activities. By doing this, there will be fewer urgent fires to take care of and therefore more time to do the items on your list!

With a regular schedule, you can arrange your time and complete all your tasks and there will be time left to grow, learn and think. We all have the same amount of time, but we just have different attitudes about it.

Some of us manage our time, other see only time constraints, (not enough time) or perhaps we see time as a liability. How we view time comes from our family, personal beliefs about ourselves, and conditioning from our outside world.

▸ Analyze how you think about time and how it should be spent. Write your thoughts about time and how you would like to change your attitudes about it.

If you find time runs away with you, learn some new skills: learn to evaluate interruptions, say *No*, schedule your time, communicate and manage stress. The more you learn to focus your time, the more productive you will be. Spend a few minutes each day planning your day and your week. Ask yourself, what are the most important things you need to accomplish this day, this week and this month?

Remember, you don't have a business until someone pays you. *Without paying clients, you just have a hobby.* Everything else is all busy work, distractions and excuses.

"Today, be aware of how you are spending your 1,440 beautiful moments, and spend them wisely." Unknown Author

When you get in overwhelm, schedule a little playtime, so that you can rejuvenate and approach your business with gusto.

▸ Spend a minute now to write down what you did yesterday (or choose a typical day). Try to remember every single thing you did.

▸ How much time did you spend contributing to your dreams?

- Did you have unaccounted time? What do you think happened to it?

- Were some of your tasks just time fillers?

- How much of this time was spent on family?

- . . . on hobbies?

- . . . on work related activities?

- . . . on marketing yourself?

- What observations do you have about your time spent yesterday?

- Spend the next few days writing down where all your time goes.

Now all this talk about time management seems to imply that I don't value quiet time. On the contrary, quiet, reflective and meditative time is very important in helping us stay focused. We all need to schedule time every day for yoga, meditation, prayer, walking, or whatever is our contemplative activity.

This time is important to our soul, and becomes an opportunity to regenerate our energy within. Our minds will let loose and find solutions to problems as we relax and focus elsewhere in nature, our breath or bodies..

Two other thoughts that will help you keep control of your time. 1.Delegate when possible. 2. Don't be a perfectionist about things that don't matter.

So, how should you spend your time? In the first stages of building your practice you should spend 80% of your available work time marketing your business.

Here's an example: You work a forty-hour week. You have five hours booked with clients and another hour for the administrative duties associated with those clients, this leaves thirty-four available hours this week. Under this scenario, twenty-seven hours should be spent on marketing!

Then of course you need time for yourself, your family and errands. No wonder you have to focus! So, how do you do this?

First, leave everything that's not important for now, if it doesn't contribute to bringing in additional clients. Then write a to-do list for later. Don't worry about outlining a benefit plan for your employee (so you are ready when you get one). The elaborate accounting system can wait, so can shopping for new office furniture. This is the time to get out and network, make phone calls, mail letters, distribute coupons, write, speak and promote yourself!

Perhaps you work from home and spend the morning cleaning house, and the afternoons running personal errands. Well, if you have children at home try to mix the car-pooling time with a run to the copy store to check on your business cards.

If you work in a shared office, do you rearrange the plants for the perfect Fung Shui, and make tea for your office mates? Offer to clean the bathroom? Perhaps you could plan a joint open house instead.

Now you know, you must spend 80% of your time working toward your dream of having paying clients, building your practice, working for yourself. And now that you know this, you have to put the plan into action.

Sometimes we lie to ourselves, insisting that we really are working our business. "I *am* working" we whine, but secretly we spend twenty hours a week reading. Yes I know they are the industry magazines, but ask yourself, if you are rationalizing your lack of time commitment with a need to *keep up* with what's going on.

Promise yourself that you will spend as much time as you can developing your practice and marketing yourself.

Perhaps it is just five hours a week that you can give. Use your lunch break from your administrative job, or work after the kids get to bed. Whatever you can do, spend that time each day and each week to building your practice. I promise you it will pay off!

▸ Ask how much time can I spend this week on promoting and building my business?

"It is an immutable law in business that words are words, explanations are explanations, promises are promises but only performance is reality." Harold S. Geneen

*I*ndividual Attributes

"You will become as small as your controlling desires, as great as your dominant aspiration." James Allen

"God gave us two ears but only one mouth. ..(perhaps) a divine indication that we should listen twice as much as we talk." John Powell

What makes an exceptional holistic practitioner? Is it one who practices wholeness? I believe it is! The exceptional therapist is one who integrates all parts of herself, allowing the polarities of life to come into balance within. As we allow life to flow through us, and we participate fully without taking any of it too seriously, we may become clear channels for our specific therapy. It is all about balance: learning to balance our lives, our sickness, our desires, our fears. All of these are just a part of who we are, until we change - and then it is no longer part of our experience. We learn to let go. To stay in balance. To learn, understand, to let go, live.

Chinese texts describe balance as *equilibrium and harmony in the body, and in life.* According to the Chinese model of medicine, having balance in your life will lead to health and healing. *Britannica* defines healing as "to restore to original purity and integrity."

The practitioners who consistently heal themselves, know that only through their own understanding of the process can they help others on the journey to wellness. As part of this restoration for you and your client, you will be working not only on physical levels of balance, but also on the mental, emotional and spiritual levels. "But wait" you say, "I already know how to be a practitioner, I just want to know how to market myself." Well, to market yourself, you must know yourself well; your strengths, weaknesses and uniqueness. If you want a successful business, you must be able to tap into the inner self and your attributes. What inner strengths can you draw from?

What? You aren't yet sure about your strengths? Relax, with time you will find your own voice and your way to connect with your clients. As you embrace all the levels of self – spiritual, emotional, physical and energetic – you will teach and learn. You will be exceptional.

Therapists always come from a compassionate and caring inner core. They genuinely care about others, and understand what the process of healing and self-discovery is like. The exceptional practitioners embrace this part of themselves and understand their clients, because they themselves have been there. They never feel as if they have arrived, but they study, continuing to learn about alternate modalities and continuing to heal themselves in all areas of their lives. They go deeper into their own expertise, whether it is nutrition, homeopathy or energy work. With continual curiosity in their own lives, they offer a deeper experience of wellness to their clients.

Exceptional practitioners incorporate many modalities, which may include homeopathy, nutrition, flower essences, intention, energy work, lifestyle changes, and creativity. They don't stop with one therapy. These practitioners are extremely intuitive and trust the process, which, in turn, strengthens their intuition even more. Exceptional therapists share the ability to listen, educate, create trust, and be a role model for the healing of others. By modeling these attributes, you will create hope for the future, hope for healing, hope for living a creative, fulfilling life.

Now, on top of all this you must run your own business, understand profit and loss statements, cash flow projections, focus on client retention, have the equivalent of a PhD in marketing, and perhaps even supervise staff! No wonder it can seem overwhelming at times! The key is to take it one step at a time, learning as you go.

Remember, being a practitioner means *practicing*.

We admire our role models not because they are perfect, but because they practice their beliefs on a daily basis. Our intuitive knowing is that they have some peace, work towards a greater life, can understand what we have been through, and can help us reach our own potential. They live each day not judging themselves or others but live from their center with healing energy. They practice healing from a mental, emotional, spiritual, physical place each day so that they may reflect this back to their clients.

Don't you hope that some qualities and characteristics of your favorite healers will rub off on you? Do you wish you were centered, balanced, focused, talented? Well of course you are! And the therapists with qualities you admire have worked to magnetize the perfect clientele to them, just as you magnetize the perfect therapist to you. We learn from each other. These therapists you admire are mirroring back to you these same qualities in yourself!

▸ Think about the following traits: discipline, confidence, spontaneity, drive, quickness, enthusiasm, patience, stamina, awareness, inquisitiveness, open-mindedness, responsiveness, creativity. Take notes as you ponder.

▸ Do you have a mentor, or a favorite practitioner? What makes them special? What qualities do they model that you admire?

▸ Which of these qualities do you have? Which would you like to develop more fully? Are some of these qualities ones you are already developing in yourself?

Here are some qualities that I admire:

▸ Commitment
▸ Integrity
▸ Trust
▸ Empathy
▸ Spiritual Guidance

We've already talked about commitment. Here's a discussion of the rest of these qualities.

23

_I_ntegrity

"Wheresoever you go, go with all your heart."
Confucius

Integrity is following though with your word.

Integrity is paying your bills and not buying something if you can't afford it.

Integrity is keeping a professional relationship with your clients (no dating!).

Integrity is staying within legal boundaries, obtaining required licenses, and paying taxes.

Integrity is living right, so your mom would be proud.

"Work is love made visible." Kahlil Gibran

Trust

"You have to have your heart in the business and the business in your heart." Thomas J. Watson

Perhaps this is obvious, but I will mention it anyway. *Always keep your client files confidential.* Always talk about case histories in general terms unless you have permission to discuss a specific client with another practitioner. Don't talk about one client to another client as this is betraying a confidence. Yes, even though and yes, even but, and yes, even if you think the client won't mind.

Once I was having an acupuncture session when the doctor turned to me and said, "You know Susan, well she was in today getting the result of her fertility testing."

I was mortified. If this were information Susan had wanted me to know, she would have told me personally. Obviously the doctor presumed I already knew about the test since we were close friends. But the doctor presumed wrong. I didn't know. And now I was in a position of knowing something Susan didn't wish me to know. And I wished I didn't. I was angry and now I had an ethical dilemma to deal with. Do I tell Susan? Do I keep my mouth shut? Do I tell my acupuncturist that in fact, I had no idea Susan was getting infertility treatments. What would you do?

Enough said. Keep your mouth shut.

*E*mpathy

"When you listen with empathy to another person, you give that person psychological air." Stephen R. Covey

I strongly believe that listening carefully to clients and caring deeply from the heart is why practitioners will retain clients. Clients expect traditional Western doctors and their office staff to be curt, hurried and poor listeners. Many patients in this model never have an opportunity to talk about their symptoms, what is changing in themselves, how they feel emotionally about aging or health concerns. The exceptional healing practitioner is a facilitator who can guide the client through a maze of often contradictory and confusing materials. They can hear what the client doesn't say, and ask the right questions.

We want to receive understanding, compassion, and clear choices when we see a practitioner. We want a shoulder to cry on and someone who cares. Alternative therapies can offer this in a way that a Western model cannot.

You can establish empathy by taking just a few minutes at the beginning of a session. First, find out how and why the client has come to you. What are her objectives? What does she hope to gain by becoming your client? Listen intently. Ask lots of questions. Take a few moments at the start of each visit to connect on a personal level. Listen with your whole body. Engage your eyes and your heart. Take time to learn how to have an exceptional, caring attitude and bedside (tableside) manner.

You have an opportunity to give unconditional listening to your clients. But know that listening is a skill that involves slowing down, paying attention and being attentive. When you listen, give it your compassionate, caring heart. Offer yourself fully in the moment and really connect with the other person. Listen with your eyes and all of your body language, as well as your ears. When you maintain eye contact you are saying that you care. Listen with understanding and ask questions if you aren't sure what is being said. Then your clients know that they are heard and understood. Help them to get their feelings, anxieties and hurts out into the open. Don't take anything for granted when you are listening. Don't assume you think you know what they will say! Allow others to speak from the heart and give them emotional space to say whatever comes up.

I'm sure you have heard "Advice unasked for is advice unappreciated." Allow the client to speak openly before you talk. If advice isn't asked for, don't give it. Don't judge your client if they haven't acted in a way you would prefer or if you feel they aren't making changes fast enough. Most of us know exactly what we need to do to make changes in our lives, but sometimes we have to talk and share our problems so that our solutions can become clear in our own mind. Treat listening as a brainstorming session for your client. Take mental notes (but not physical notes – yet) Listen in such a way that the friend or client can be totally open and feel absolutely free to share his or her deepest need without being judged. Take notes on paper after your client has finished sharing, and take notes as appropriate to your modality and as it relates to your session. Remember to keep everything confidential!

Mary Kay Ash, founder of Mary Kay Cosmetics, said that the secret to success was making believe that every person you're speaking with is wearing a sign around their neck that says, "Make me feel important!" One of the most basic human needs is to feel valued and it should be your goal to make each and every client feel that they're special and number one.

As you begin to know your clients they will reveal their inner motivations and create intimacy and trust in your relationship. They will heal faster and you will be rewarded by your professionalism and repeat business. You will feel gratified by helping others.

The exceptional practitioner offers acceptance of their clients, no matter where they are on their journey, and then they meet them there, at that place of readiness, wherever that may be.

Not every client is ready, able or willing to be on the caffeine-free, sugar-free, white flour-free diet along with a regimen of exercising and mediating every day. Find some common ground, a place to meet your client halfway.

What are your clients willing to do? Start there. Build trust. Get to know them. Then, stretch them as fast and as far as they can go (but not so fast that they may break and never come back to see you again)!

Some, of course, will embrace everything you suggest, walking the straight and healthful path of great nutrition, daily walks, supplementation and massage. For others, cutting out just one soda per day will be enough for them to start on their journey.

Bill, a naturopath, felt so strongly about his nutrition regimen, he asked every new client to sign a contract listing their new diet requirements. He didn't even want to work with clients if they weren't totally committed to change. Did this work for him? Well, he got exactly the type of client base he wanted - *gung ho*, serious, and focused on healing, a small base of clients that believed in him wholeheartedly, but he also turned away many others who would have started with him on a slower journey.

Be empathetic, gently guide your clients over time toward a holistic lifestyle, and applaud them for changes they can make now. Don't judge – guide and direct.

Reassure them that we all get where we are going, in our own time.

"The essence of health is trusting yourself, your thoughts, and your feelings. Self-trust is the ability to know the truth about what you think and feel in your very bones- and then to use this information to guide your life".
Christiane Northrup

Spiritual Guidance

"The unique personality which is the real life in me, I can not gain unless I search for the real life, the spiritual quality, in others." Felix Adler

Spiritual guidance has nothing to do with your religious beliefs. We have all heard the statement "When the student is ready, the teacher will appear." Often the teacher appears within us. We become our own teachers when we listen to the small voice inside telling us how to continue with our lives, which way to turn, which path to choose.

I've noticed that some practitioners have an ability to let go, to detach at the right moments, and then to hang on for dear life at other times. Their timing is impeccable. They listen to the small voice within and trust it.

This inner guidance is a strength that combines all the above qualities with experience and preparation. It is knowing that there is nothing to fear. We embrace all of life and take it as it comes. We express our emotions and don't apologize for them, but neither do we become attached to them. We realize it too, will pass.

Inner strength can come from knowing you have something to offer *just because you are you.*

▸ What can you do to strongly develop your intuition and your own spiritual guidance within yourself?

"Grace is available for each of us every day — our spiritual daily bread — but we've got to remember to ask for it with a grateful heart and not worry about whether there will be enough for tomorrow." Sarah Ban Breathnach

Financial Abundance

"The world is full of abundance and opportunity, but far too many people come to the fountain of life with a sieve instead of a tank car, a teaspoon instead of a steam shovel. They expect little and as a result they get little."
Ben Sweetland

We all want to live in abundance. We learn that financial abundance is available for us if only we would have the right positive outlook and confidence that we deserve it. In other words, the cash is ours if we trust in the Universe.

Our teachers have told us that if we have lived in a poverty mentality we should now be ready to shake the old attitudes, and then God, (and the Universe) will support us.

Yes, we must have a huge amount of faith – faith in ourselves, faith in God, faith in our training, faith that the Universe will provide for us. Yet we must also go out in the world, do the work, learn how to run our businesses, market ourselves, and get on with co–creating our lives.

Perhaps you've heard that old saying, "Trust in God but tie up your horse." It's not enough to sit back and take whatever comes, believing that our attitudes alone will bring in the money.

Of course this is partially true – our attitudes will have a great deal to do with our abundance, but we must also back it up with our actions.

We do have to have a strong belief system. We believe with a deep knowing inside self (different from just wishing it was so) and then, after we have that knowingness and faith within us, we must go do the work to make it all happen.

We want to have great attitudes, live in abundance mentality and expect the best, but we also have to find our clients, charge for our services and then, the most important step ever, accept payment!

- ▸ Examine how you feel about money? Ashamed? Proud? Scared?

- How are your cash management skills?

- Can you balance a checkbook?

- Pay your bills on time?

- Manage a credit card without getting into debt?

- Can you blow a bundle and never know what you did with it?

However you choose to manage your cash, take control of it. Be comfortable with managing it; after all, it is one of your great resources. Understand how it affects your life and your power.

Budgeting, learning to conserve and treating ourselves to luxuries on occasion, can help our mental well-being and sense of control.

If we feel powerless over money, then the money will have power over us.

Still, having power over money doesn't mean being obsessed with it, but it does mean being comfortable enough to manage our cash wisely. Learn to be a friend with your money.

Cash, of course, is just one level of currency in your life.

Julia Cameron, in *The Artist's Way*, talks about money this way: "All too often we become blocked and blame it on our lack of money. This is never an authentic block. The actual block is our feeling of constriction, our sense of powerlessness. Art requires us to empower ourselves with choice. At the most basic level, this means choosing to do self–care."

Now you may not be an artist, but the point remains clear. As we become blocked, we blame all our ills on our lack of cash. We feel as though the money is controlling our lives, when really all we should be doing is taking better care of ourselves. We should be looking within to satisfy our needs. Once we meet those needs by taking care of ourselves, our addictions to money can come into balance. Then we can use money as a way to negotiate safely around the world.

- Do you have struggles with money, or a belief that having money is shallow, selfish or somehow wrong?

- Then enroll in a cash management class.

- Ask the bank to teach you to balance your checkbook.

- Learn how to invest. Knowledge is power.

- Take a moment now and write again about money.

Does writing about it bring up feelings for you? Allow your subconscious to process your thoughts without analyzing them.

"The abundant life does not come to those who have had a lot of obstacles removed from their path by others. It develops from within and is rooted in strong mental and moral fiber."
William Mather Lewis

Pricing Our Services

"I did toy with the idea of doing a cook–book. .
. . I think a lot of people who hate literature but love fried
eggs would buy it if the price was right." Groucho Marx

Cathy has said she wishes she could give away her services. She feels bad charging for healing other people. "I only want to help others" she moans, when we talk about how much she charges. She tells me she wants to live her life in service to others.

Of course she wants to be in service. Life is most rewarding when we can help others. If you are reading this book you probably have already devoted your life to healing others. If you picked up this book you also want to increase your income. You want to be in service and also financially secure.

You must get used to the idea that you can charge a fair price and then collect the money. You just can't give away your services for free. You have overhead, bills, families and responsibilities. Even if you *are* financially secure without a care in the world about money, you should still charge unless you build your practice totally around charity to others. For the rest of us, money is the accepted and expected exchange.

Don't feel bad about having to charge for your services. Some in the healing community believe there should be no charge for healing or spiritual services; however, we must be realistic about our own physical needs. The money we earn we can also spend and that helps the world go 'round!

Being realistic and honest with ourselves keeps us in integrity. If we offer our services to others at almost no charge, this may force us to be out of integrity with our own financial obligations.

What is a realistic budget based upon your obligations and needs? Below, list your financial requirements so that you can see on paper the expectations you must have.

▸   Here is a small sample home budget, fill in your own numbers:

Business Cards/Brochures/Flyers

Cable

Car Maintenance and Gasoline

Car Payment

Car Insurance

Clothing

Computer

Entertainment

Food

Health Costs (insurance co–pay, etc)

Household

Insurance Business

Insurance Home

Internet Services/email/web site & maintenance

Loan Payments

Office Supplies

Personal Items

Phone Home

Phone Business

Postage

Rent Business

Rent /House payment

Trade Publications

Trade Shows

Utilities Business

Utilities Home

Other

Other

Other

Income:

Income from other sources:

▸ Do you see your expenses more clearly? What thoughts do you have?

So, how should you charge for your services? Start by conducting your own market research. What do others charge for a session? Pricing yourself competitively in the middle of the range is a good place to start.

Consider these questions when setting your price.

- Are your sessions hourly?
- Do you charge per session or per hour?
- Are your sessions the same length as your peers?
- Can you make longer or shorter sessions, adapting to clients' needs and then price accordingly?
- Do you offer unique touches that you can charge for? (i.e., herbal teas, hot towels, relaxation time)
- If you price yourself lower, will they perceive you as *less than*?
- If you price yourself higher, will they perceive you as *more than*?

When setting your price, keep in mind that you can always offer special promotions, coupons and discounts to lower your rate; however raising your rates is difficult.

When offering discounts, package them to encourage customer loyalty. Here are some ideas you can discuss with your clients:

- Bring in a friend for a 25% discount.
- Purchase (and pay for!) five sessions up front and receive a special package price.
- Refer five people, get a free session.
- Book a double session for a discount.
- Schedule six months of sessions and get a free *goody basket*.

Or perhaps you could:

- Offer gift certificates with an extra 15 minutes session time. Allow your regular clients to purchase these for themselves.
- Give away lotions, oils, gifts on birthdays or after 10 sessions.

The point is to be creative and reward your regular clients.

All that said, you might safely donate up to 10% of your time if you choose.

"The more we learn to operate in the world based on trust in our intuition, the stronger our channel will be and the more money we will have." Shakti Gawain

*M*arketing, so what is it anyway?

"Being busy does not always mean real work. The object of all work is production or accomplishment and to either of these ends there must be forethought, system, planning, intelligence and honest purpose, as well as perspiration. Seeming to do, is not doing." Thomas Edison

For many of us marketing is an overwhelming idea involving advertising and selling, business plans and market analysis. We believe we have to sell ourselves and push our products onto people who don't want them. Repeatedly I hear; "I don't like to sell myself, I just wish someone else would do the selling for me. I don't even have to make too much money, just enough so that I can continue serving others."

The image of a typical salesperson is loud, obnoxious and unconscious of themselves and others. They manipulate others to get what they want and sell us something we don't need. We know that advertising is costly and anyway, it usually involves a teenage girl in scantily dressed clothes. Ick! Who wants to be a part of all that?

In a perfect world, our clients would miraculously magnetize themselves to us and we'd wait by the phone and take appointments. Unfortunately, that rarely works. Yes we need to put ourselves and our services *out there* – but the good news is we *can* magnetize others who value our services. The key to this is to understand that *marketing is nothing more than building relationships.* When you build on a relationship and the customer has a chance to feel in control, they won't feel manipulated or pushed into a sale.

Marketing yourself involves everything you do to sell yourself and build your business. This includes being clear about your business, behaving professionally, connecting with others in a one-on-one or networking situation, living with integrity, and providing exceptional customer service.

You are marketing yourself when you print a business card or introduce yourself to someone new. Marketing includes booking the next appointment for a present client as well as calling to follow up when you haven't heard from a client in a while. Marketing is everything you do to connect with others.

When we buy something, especially a service, it is our emotion that dictates how we spend our money, not reason. We buy from someone because we like them and we will only buy if it makes us feel good.

We use an astrologer or psychic or therapist because we feel affirmed, hopeful, enlightened or healed in some way after the session. We feel good about the person and the service. After a session, we want our feelings to be confirmed and feel that we made the right decision.

Marketing and selling a service is very different from selling a product. When you sell a product, the customer can pick up something tangible, then smell, see, touch and evaluate it. Selling a service means selling *yourself* and building trust before a client will use your service. Your clients are buying a complete package that is you. This includes your training, your unique approach, outlook, image, personality and skills.

Clients want to get to know their therapist personally. It is your unique personality that causes a client to choose you over another practitioner. How you present yourself is the core of your marketing thrust.

If you think about building your practice by creating relationships with others, you will find your practice will grow quickly and with the least amount of work. All you will do is to meet new people, take care of existing clients and nurture the relationships you currently have.

Yes, it will take some effort, but the effort won't seem like work. It will be a natural extension of your healing gifts.

So where do you network and meet people to get these new clients? Well, where have you gotten your past clients?

• List five of your clients. How did they first hear about you? Where did they come from?

This is the first step in marketing. – Keeping track of what is working for you and recording it.

Review your whole client list now. Can you remember how each of them became a client?

‣ Write down any more referral sources.

When Joanne, a client of mine, first did this exercise, she realized that most of her clients came from referrals and most of the referrals came from just one person. With this new knowledge, she is able to back to this person and ask for more referrals – obviously a technique that works for her. She also asked other clients for referrals and started a reward program that included free Reiki sessions and homemade gift baskets.

From now on, ask each client how they heard about you. What made them choose you? What was the catalyst? Keep track of this information so that you can see what works and how it changes.

- Start a marketing plan!

Purchase a small notebook to hold all the information from these exercises. Continue to add to this notebook over the years so that you can track your progress, evaluate what is working for you, plan your efforts and then work your plan!

When practitioners start a new business in, say, massage or astrology, the questions they always ask are, where do I start? How do I get clients? Should I advertise in the yellow pages? Should I get an office, phone and business cards first, or advertise first? The quick answer is you are going to do it all, but slowly, inexpensively and with careful thought.

One of the first steps is to do a little market research.

- Ask your current clients (friends and family will work) why they come to see you as a practitioner.

What is it they like about your services? If they had to find a new practitioner, what would they look for? Have they ever been to one of your competitors or peers? What did they like or dislike about the service?

Ask yourself these same questions.

- Who do you choose to see for service in your same profession?

- Why? What if you need to find a new hairdresser, doctor or babysitter, how would you start searching for the perfect person?

Perhaps location is important to you, but to your mother, a relaxing environment with chamomile tea is the most important. Why do clients buy your service and how do they choose it?

As an example, my friend RuthAnne has a roaring massage business. How does she keep a full schedule? Well, clients, including me, like her because she offers several services. Massage, cranial, deep tissue, somatic movement, spiritual counseling; there is a large bag of skills to draw from and she uses them all. She always asks if I would like to book my next appointment before I leave her office. Then, as I leave, RuthAnne schedules the day and time, handing me a card with my new appointment date.

Cindee, who is a full time freelance writer, builds her business through marketing herself. She tells everyone she meets that she can write for all types of publications. When asked, she estimates she still spends 80% of her time marketing, sending out query letters, following up with editors and magazines, and researching new places to write.

Cindee has been writing full time for several years and still spends the bulk of her time marketing herself. What has changed, however, is the amount of money she now earns per word. Cindee is paid a lot, but it wasn't that way in the beginning. Now her writing is in demand and she still writes every day. Puts pen to paper and gets it done. She writes. And then markets what she writes. Every day.

This is how it must be with you. Every day, get up and market yourself. Do a little of your craft, see some clients and market yourself some more. Talk to your clients before they leave your office. Can you book your client for the rest of the year on a regular schedule? Can you sell them a gift certificate?

Do you clients know about other services you offer? Chair massage? On-call for home visits? Do they have a friend they can recommend you to?

Start now and soon marketing yourself will become automatic and then you too will be able to raise your prices.

"Business has only two functions – marketing and innovation." Peter F. Drucker

A dvertising

"As to the idea that advertising motivates people, remember the Edsel." Peter Drucker

A personal thought about advertising.

Don't do it. At least not yet. Not until you can afford to spend the cash and you already have started to establish a name for yourself. Advertising rarely brings in new customers in this industry. It will simply keep your name in front of your customers and build on your reputation.

A polarity therapist called to ask me whether to take out a Yellow Page ad. I asked her when was the last time she chose a therapist from the Yellow Pages? In years of consulting I have never found these ads to work unless the therapist already has built their reputation.

Yes, you may get a few calls from the yellow pages and perhaps even a few clients, but do the math first. How much per month do you have to spend for the few calls you are likely to get. Will the ad pay for itself?

Therapists get clients by word of mouth and keep them through excellent customer service. This is true with few exceptions.

Of course there are exceptions. Of course there are times when you should advertise.

Perhaps you are writing an article for a local business publication. Then, please, take a small advertisement alongside the article to help promote yourself.

If you participate in a trade show, take out an ad in the brochure to help promote your booth.

Do you have a local health related magazine? Advertise to support networking efforts.

See how this works? Advertise to support your ongoing efforts, not to replace them. Consider offering promotions or discounts to new clients. Reevaluate your advertising every six months and search for new opportunities. Always, before advertising, do the math to see if you will recoup your investment.

*C*larity

"For me the greatest beauty always lies in the greatest clarity." **Gotthold Lessing**

"Take advantage of every opportunity to practice your communication skills so that when important occasions arise, you will have the gift, the style, the sharpness, the clarity and the emotions to affect other people." **Jim Rohn**

In this section the exercises will ask you for inner reflection of your self, your practice and your image. In going through the exercises you will begin to sort through information that helps define who you are and how you present yourself. You have probably thought about most of this before, but write it down anyway. You will find a pattern of your inner beliefs will emerge. Writing will help you clarify your thoughts. You will begin to understand your own motivations so that each time you talk with someone, or write a flier, it will come from the same inner voice.

This chapter explores the following questions.

- Do you have a ten second introduction for yourself?

- Can you explain your service in clear, concise terms your service?

- Do you know what your business stands for?

- What benefits do you offer clients?

- Where would you like your practice to be in a year?

For the most part, clients will choose a therapist, not the therapy. Be clear about what you offer and what it is that makes you different from other therapists so you can stand apart from them.

▸ Evaluate your own decision–making process for visiting other service professionals. How do you make your choices when choosing a new hairdresser, therapist or health care provider?

What is important to you? Training? Location? Personality? Cleanliness?

▸ Why do you continue to see the same providers while you never go back to others?

The reasons that you choose providers are some of the same reasons clients will use when they choose you.

▸ What are some reasons you would *not* return to a provider?

For instance, too chatty, not chatty enough, poor location, a dirty restroom, lack of skill, runs late for appointments. Write your top ten reasons. Again, be specific.

"Life is a field of unlimited possibilities"
Deepak Chopra

*F*eatures and Benefits

"I don't know the key to success, but the key to failure is trying to please everybody." Bill Cosby

Now, after all this talk of selling ourselves, I take it all back. You aren't selling yourself at all, but you are selling the *benefit* of your therapy..

It's the personal stuff that matters to us and our clients. We want to know what's in it for us? Why do we care? We want to know how it will help us. You need simple concise language for your client to understand what you do and how it will benefit them right here, right now.

The key to marketing yourself is to take your features and explain them as benefits. It is important to differentiate between the two.

Mike, a massage therapist, is a client who came to me for help in building his business. He has been a therapist for a little over a year and didn't know how to expand his practice. I asked him to explain to me what he did.

"Well," he said, "I've been trained in all types of massage. Swedish, deep tissue, relaxation, hot rocks, you name it, I can do it. At my last job at the spa, my bosses gave us classes in aroma therapy and essential oils. I feel I have all the skills it takes to be successful."

In Mike's case, the features are his training in several types of bodywork, aroma therapy and essential oils. These will all be helpful in creating his unique marketing approach. Yet Mike has to tell us why it matters to us and as the client, we want to know what's in it for us.

For instance, because of his extensive training and experience, one of his skills is to tune into a new client, and within moments, read the body and choose an appropriate therapy and oil. Mike can then talk about how wonderful the room will smell and how our body will respond to the oils. His knowledge (features) can be translated into benefits.

Your feature might be the type of training, the degree or certificate you have, who trained you and your years of experience. The key is to turn that into a benefit for the clients by telling (or showing) them why they should care. If you have had twenty–seven years of training in twelve different modalities I need to know why that will help me. Explain how your experience translates into a benefit for me, the client.

Zoe has been a massage therapist for almost twenty years. She has taken classes in many types of herbal remedies, essential oils and flower essences. When she talks about herself, she accentuates her expertise in helping clients move through emotional issues quickly using this expanded knowledge.

She finds clients move through emotional issues in just a few sessions, *even if they have been working on these issues for years!* She's not just talking about her training, she tells us how we benefit.

The feature is about you. The benefit is about your client.

Find the benefits in these sentences below:

- Whatever stress or complaint you have, I feel confident that my energy work can align your Chakras so that you will feel more balanced and focused by the time you leave my office.

- I promptly sense the type of work your body will respond to and will help you relax immediately.

- Since I've spent years studying, I won't have to spend your time looking up oils in the reference books. Together we can choose the oils that will work with your ailments and help you feel more energized.

- My pressure can be gentle or strong depending upon your mood.

- I have highly–developed intuition and I can hone in on hidden problem areas.

- The drive is well worth it. It's so quiet out here in the country that you will start relaxing on the drive out and have time to unwind before you reenter the city. Everyone loves coming out and so will you.

- I love working with people's nervous systems and I'm an expert in using the natural rhythms of the body. I'll focus on you and let your body show me the way it wants to work. We can get more done in less time this way.

- Did you know there is fluid that runs up and down the body? I can feel that fluid and help the body in directing its own flow. When we are done, you'll feel as though you were ten years younger!

One way to write out a feature/benefit sentence is to say what it is you do (take one example), and then, what it does for the client.

For instance,

- What I do is massage; the reason you care is that it will make your body feel good!

- What I do is balance your Chakras; the reason you care is that it will help you get in touch with your spiritual self and help you be centered and calm.

▸   Finish the following:

What I do is,

You care because,

Another way to approach features and benefits is to imagine you are explaining how to fix a certain problem. I'll demonstrate using the words, "you know how_____.and well, what I do is_____."

For instance, you know how your lower back gets tight and sore after gardening? Well, what I do is release the muscles so they can relax. You'll feel better instantly!

▸   Try this for yourself:

You know how . . .

Well, what I do is . . .

"If he was to become himself, he must find a way to assemble the parts of his dreams into one whole." George Eliot

M^{otivation}

> **"In my experience, there is only one motivation and that is desire. No reasons or principle contain it or stand against it."**
> *Jane Smiley*

Your inner motivation is a key to marketing effectively. As you examine your motives, they will surface and you will connect with others who resonate with you. The same motives that attract you will attract others.

Write some quick stream-of-consciousness answers to the questions below. Some questions that follow may seem similar, but I have designed them to help you access deeper answers within yourself. With the information gathered below, you'll start formulating your introduction and written materials, bringing it together.

- What do you love about the specific therapy you practice?

- Why did you get started in this business?

- What do you give to your clients? Calling to ask them may be valuable! It is often surprising what people will tell us when we ask.

- What is it you want your clients to say about you?

Ok. I'm going to make some assumptions now. Who are your present clients? Probably mostly women, aged 30–60 looking for a change in their lives. Often these women are looking for peace, clarity and physical comfort or just want to be pampered. These women have tried many different modalities, with some success, but perhaps not in the holistic realm. (If you have men and children in your practice, they may have been referred by a woman in their lives, or by another practitioner).

- Who are your clients now? Be specific in your answer, age, gender, income, race, location, interests.

Notice what they may all have in common.

Can you specialize within the above client base? For instance, can you work more closely with some menopausal women or in prenatal care?

Using the information from above, write a paragraph answering the following questions.

- Who is your target market?

- What type of person uses your service?

- What motivates someone to use your service?

Your Uniqueness

"While we have the gift of life, it seems to me the only tragedy is to allow part of us to die — whether it is our spirit, our creativity or our glorious uniqueness."
Gilda Radner

What makes you different from everyone else in your field? Is it location? Philosophy? Why do your clients come to you? Perhaps you specialize? What about your own background? Story? Training? How do your clients resonate with you?

► Write a brief statement showing why you are unique. Include your, philosophy, location, education, specialties and anything else that comes to mind.

I^{mage}

"A strong, positive self–image is the best possible preparation for success." *Joyce Brothers*

Your image consists of many things: dress, presentation, professionalism, experience, location, the energy you exude. It includes everything that makes people think of you in a certain way. Do you have integrity? Personal ethics and a fair understanding of customer service? Does your outward appearance coincide with your inner desires?

How would you like to be thought of in your community? What strengths would you like to develop?

Perhaps you are laid back, a relaxed person who gets along with everyone. Does your image and business reflect that?

Maybe you are a go–getter, eager to build up a reputation as one who can help others achieve their goals. Do your dress, style and reputation help you mirror that image?

▸ Write a brief statement about the image you would like to portray.

▸ How close is the desired image of your self to the image you are portraying right now?

▸ What steps can you take today to help these two come together?

Your introduction

"Do not become paralyzed and enchained by the set patterns which have been woven of old. No, build from your own youthful feeling, your own groping thought and your own flowering perception . . . " Lotte Lehmann

By now you have a wealth of information that you can draw upon to write an introduction. Go back and read through all your answers thus far and use them as you write an introduction for yourself. Don't worry about how it sounds, just get it down on paper. Allow your subconscious to take the next few days to sort it out. The next time you introduce yourself, it will be a well thought out presentation!

▸ Write an introduction and include your name, the features and benefits, (what you do and why the client cares), your specialties, who your clients are and what makes you unique.

*P*romotional Materials

"We are the products of editing, rather than authorship." George Wald

We need written promotional materials including business cards, brochures and fliers, but we get bogged down and in overwhelm when it comes to designing and writing them.

The next few pages will outline a template to help you write your own brochures and other written materials.

▸ The first thing to do is to collect business cards, brochures and fliers from other therapists.

Get everything. The ones you like and ones that you don't. You can collect them from any industry, but collect only materials that market a service.

Lay all these items in front of you on a large table. At first glance, put them into two piles. The ones that appeal and the ones that don't.

What do you notice about the ones you like? Is it the material? Color? Font? Do you like the specific layouts or designs of certain business cards?

Do the same analysis of the materials that don't appeal and then toss those aside for now. You can always go back to them later. Return to the appealing pile. Pull out a few of your favorites and read them. Notice if you like simple designs, full bright color, or certain layouts. Is there a particular card or brochure that would prompt you to call and follow up with this person? Why?

▸ Take a few notes about the things you like and dislike about the materials.

The local office supply store has a stock selection of business cards and brochures from which to choose. There are several very pleasant low cost designs.

You can also purchase low–cost business cards to get you started. A word of warning though, choose a heavy card stock for business cards. The flimsy cards look and feel cheap and won't help you promote an image of well-being in your practice.

I recommend printing only a minimum amount of materials and printing on your own computer if possible. Sometimes clients will print 500 cards, (usually the minimum available from a printer) and then have corrections or additions within a few weeks. Print the minimum you can start with, maybe 50 or so cards, and try them out for a few weeks before stocking up.

Have a trusted friend, (or two!) proofread all your written materials before going to press and don't be too surprised if some mistake slips through. It usually does.

Business Cards

"I decided that I would be one of the biggest new names and I actually had some little fancy business cards printed up to announce it. Beware, the Count is Here."
Count Basie

Everyone needs a business card. It is your introduction to the world and conveys your image and service to others quickly. Business cards are a great marketing tool because they staying around. They rarely get thrown out and so they are part of your low cost ongoing marketing effort. It is your first written contact with the world and can be used as a mini brochure or flier.

You can print cards in any direction. Try one or two-sided, use a folded card with information on the inside, or a postcard instead of a standard business card size. You can use the backside to write appointment dates on.

Make sure the card represents who you are and feels energetically like you. You have to feel proud when you give out your card as you'll be carrying them everywhere and passing them out at every opportune moment. This is the fastest, easiest way to get your name and business out to the community.

So, how to write your cards? Include your complete name, address, business name or title and phone number. Try to incorporate a brief sentence describing your service.

- Low–cost massage – at your home!
- Chakra balancing for spiritual well–being

Remember to include your zip code and area code. Business cards have a way of traveling out of town, so you may get a referral from a visiting friend. The point is to make sure you are reachable!

If you choose not to include an address, think about renting a post office box so that you can receive mail from others. You will want to receive mail about promotions, trade show opportunities, open houses and other networking events.

Brochures, fliers and such

"Come to the edge," He said. They said, "We are afraid." "Come to the edge," He said. They came. He pushed them... and they flew. Guillaume Apollinaire

Your brochure should be an invitation for a prospective client to telephone you, ask for more information, or to book an appointment. The main objective of a brochure is to stir up interest so that a prospect will phone you! A brochure can be many places at once, doing the marketing for you. Post your brochure on bulletin boards, in offices, and in waiting rooms. Get your name out there! Your goal should be to have your name familiar to others in the community. In time, your prospective clients will have seen your name so much that they will feel as though they already know you!

A brochure should clearly reflect who you are as a person, what your strengths are, features, benefits and what you offer. Write your brochure in clear concise language, free of industry jargon.

Brochures can be one page or multiple pages, and almost any size and shape. It is easiest to print on 81/2 x 11 paper and fold it in half or thirds. Keep in mind that the brochure will speak for you, anticipate and answer certain questions, educate potential clients and ask them to contact you.

Here are a few simple rules to keep in mind when designing a brochure.

- Leave lots of white space. Don't fill the paper with too much text as it can be difficult to read.

- Use bullets or lists to make your key points.

- Choose one or two font types only.

- Keep the type size consistent.

- Include testimonials – recommendations from others.

- Incorporate a call to action – perhaps a coupon.

- Include features and benefits.

- Have your contact information complete.

- Include expiration dates when applicable.

When writing the text of your brochure ask these questions:

- Who? What? When? Where? Why? How?

This information will make the brochure flow and assure you include all the pertinent information. By following this simple template, you will be able to write any promotional material with ease.

- Who am I? –My credentials.

- Who is the client? –Audience.

- What do I do? The feature.

- What will the client get? The benefit.

- When should they come? When they hurt? Or every month for maintenance?

- When are you open? Your hours and days of operation.

- Where are you? Location, mine or yours?

- Why are you a practitioner? What is your passion?

- Why should a client come? More benefits.

- What are your techniques?

- How do they make an appointment?

Finish with a call to action. The prospective client should read your brochure and be motivated to call you. What incentive can you give them? Is there a coupon attached with an expiration date? Ask them to do something that inspires them to act – to call now, to mail in something, or to book an appointment. Remember to ask them to do it.

liers

". . . in dreams begins responsibility." **Edna O'Brien**

You should use a flier when you have a special event to promote. It could be a class, open house or a one-time occasion. All of these events work well on a flier. Concentrate on only one event per flier.

The main difference between a brochure and flier is that a brochure is a general, long term, marketing tool introducing yourself and your services. A flier promotes a specific event and has an expiration date. Brochures are usually meant to be kept and are printed on nice paper. Fliers are usually made to be thrown away relatively quickly.

Fliers, like postcards, can be mailed to prospective clients two to four weeks before an event, inviting them to attend. Ask for a response so that you know how well your flier is working and how many people to expect.

Post your fliers in health food stores, bulletin boards, grocery stores, coffee shops, waiting rooms and everywhere you can think of!

When designing a flier, use bright colors – yellow and green seem to have the best response. (Lilac is the worst received color for a flier).

". . . as one goes through life one learns that if you don't paddle your own canoe, you don't move." Katharine Hepburn

Testimonials

"'Tis so much joy! 'Tis so much joy! If I should fail, what poverty! And yet, as poor as I Have ventured all upon a throw; Have gained! Yes! Hesitated so this side the victory!" Emily Dickinson

Nothing sells like a personal referral. You can use direct quotes in your marketing materials to help add impact to your presentation. Testimonials will also help alleviate the fear of the unknown. Your prospective clients will think, "Well, if So and So had a good experience, then I will too!"

Here are some examples.

"For the first time ever I have a brochure! Thanks so much! Your template helped me get it together." Suzie, Reiki Practitioner, Oregon

"I used a lot of the marketing tips in this book. After only a few months I was able to reach my goal. I never thought I'd work full time, but now my appointment book is full weeks ahead. Thank you." Michele, Holistic Medicine Specialist, Colorado

"I recommend this book to anyone wanting to start a practice. It is full of great tips." Mike, Life Coaching, Kansas

Or you could start your sentence with,

"My clients tell me that after a session they . . . "

▸ Call your three best clients and ask for a written testimonial.

*P*ress Releases

"... focus on the journey, not the destination. Joy is found not in finishing an activity but in doing it."
Greg Anderson

Press releases are great self-promotion and they are free! Use press releases to let your community know about upcoming events, accomplishments and awards, almost anything you can think of that would be of interest to others. Pick up copies of all the newspapers in your area and read the press releases that they publish. Often they will be in the business or community section of your newspaper. One afternoon, contact each paper and ask for their press release submission guidelines. You have a great chance of getting some free publicity if you just take the time to send in your news.

Here is a sample press release:

Michelle A. Vandepas
1120 Rock Creek Canyon Road
Colorado Springs CO 80926
mav@usa.net
719-527-1404

The Gazette
30 S. Prospect St.
Colorado Springs, CO 80903

October 13, 2003

For Immediate Release:

Marketing for the Holistic Practitioner Workshop is being held Saturday November 22, 2003 from 9:00 AM – Noon, at the East Branch Library. Cost is $25.00 and includes herbal teas and snacks. Call 719–527–1404 for more information.

_____

Please print this release in your weekly calendar section. If you have any questions regarding this release, please call Michelle Vandepas, 719–527–1404. Thank you.

There are many types of press releases and many articles and books written on techniques for getting press releases printed. Start simple and learn as you go!

Some ideas for press releases:

- moving your office

- an open house

- a class you are offering

- an award you received

- any special accomplishment

- an anniversary party

- offer a free seminar

The guidelines for writing a good press release:

- Keep it to a maximum of one page unless more is absolutely necessary.

- Tell about your service in one or two clear sentences.

- Create an angle of interest to the community.

- Use a great title or headline .

- Use active verbs.

- Use timely information and tie it into current events.

- Send your release to radio, TV stations, and newspapers and to your mailing list. Add Internet sites if applicable.

- Include your contact information: e-mail, Name, Address, Phone, Fax, Website.

Networking

"Decide to Network; Use every letter you write; Every conversation you have; Every meeting you attend; To express your fundamental beliefs and dreams; Affirm to others the vision of the world you want; Network through thought; Network through action; Network through love; Network through spirit; You are the center of a network; You are the center of the world; You are a free, immensely powerful source of life and goodness; Affirm it; Spread it; Radiate it; And you will see a miracle happen: the greatness of life. In a world of big powers, media, and monopolies, But of four and a half billion individuals, Networking is the new freedom, the new democracy, a new form of happiness."   Robert Muller

Selling yourself is nothing more than networking and connecting with others!

Practitioners usually hate to sell. They love what they do, their craft, but repeatedly I hear them complain about the selling. Sandra told me, "I don't want to push people into buying, I want them to just call and make an appointment. They'll know if it's right for them."

Unfortunately, Sandra sits in her spotlessly clean office waiting for the phone to ring, but she continues to have open slots in her calendar. If this sounds like you, here is your answer: Networking!

What if you were in a new town and desperately needed a massage therapist, how would you go about finding one? Perhaps you would call a health food store and ask them for a referral. Or maybe you'd call a spa and chat awhile about the therapists they offer. Maybe you'd just wait awhile and ask around. These are all a form of networking.

Networking is nothing more than meeting people, gathering connections, getting involved in your community and then using the contacts when appropriate. Selling is meeting people, listening to what they have to say, telling them what you do, and making an appointment.

In the traditional sales world, trainers teach salespeople to find an interest level, to listen intently for buying signals, overcome objections, ask for the order and then close the sale. When using networking as our sales model, this translates into: talking to people, answering their questions, offering information and asking if they would like to make an appointment. Put this way it sounds a lot less intimidating! This simple, but extremely effective technique, can be the cornerstone of your marketing efforts.

When meeting someone new, listen carefully to what is being said, and listen attentively so that you can also intuit what is not being said. Then ask questions. Lots of them. Be friendly and concerned. For instance, if you are hearing a story about someone who never uses holistic therapies, ask why... Did they have a bad experience? Are they fearful of the unknown? Do they think that holistic healing conflicts with their spiritual or religious beliefs? If you ask the questions, you can appropriately reply to their response and then overcome their concerns.

By now, you have at the very least an outline of your ten-second introduction in clear, concise terms. You have the beginnings of a brochure and business card. The next step is to bring it together and use these tools. Now is the time to get out and meet people!

Networking groups

"A am realistic -- I expect miracles."

Wayne Dyer

So where do you start? Call the library. They will have a list of all the groups in town that meet regularly. These may include women's groups, volunteer opportunities, LEADS (specifically for generating sales), and business meetings such as the Chamber of Commerce functions and the Better Business Bureau. These groups often hold meetings in local restaurants, business locations or hotels and are often scheduled at breakfast or lunch.

Groups always welcome new members. However, you shouldn't join anything yet. In the next month, go visit as many of them as you can. There is usually no charge the first time you go but be sure to ask. Just show up, introduce yourself and hand out a business card. Don't worry if you are shy, go anyway. Most people are shy the first few times they are in a new situation.

Volunteer to help set up or break down the meeting; pass out nametags, and help with registration. If you have a task, it will keep you focused and you won't be so shy. Come early. Stay late. Your goal is to meet people.

Before you go to an event wear your nametag (often they will provide them for you, but if not, make your own). Pin or clip it to your right side, so when you shake a person's hand, their eyes are led down your arm to your name.

Wear clothes with pockets to collect and receive business cards easily. Fill one pocket with business cards and your pen. During the event, put down your purse, clothes and food. Keep your hands free so that you can shake hands and pass out cards.

As you first walk into the room, see if there is a registration table or a host that welcomes newcomers. Ask if there are any other first-timers. If so, walk right up to them and introduce yourself. After all, they will feel awkward and shy too. If there aren't newcomers, find someone else to walk up to and hold out your hand. Shake hands firmly, very slightly squeezing the other person's hand. Grasp the hand fully and straight on. No limp fingers or over zealous shakes please! (Turning your hand so that your palm faces down in the handshake transmits dominance. Turning your palm up shows submission to others. Grasping only the fingers and not the whole palm shows lack of respect and/or superiority to others. A limp handshake shows lack of confidence.)

Go right up to and say, "Hi, my name is . . . and it's my first time here." Introduce yourself, and exchange business cards. Be friendly, smile, and don't worry if you are nervous, do it anyway! You have just started your network of prospective clients!

As you take their card, remember something about this person and the conversation. Ask questions, and try to put the other person at ease so that it will take the focus off you. Write some notes on the back of their card so you remember them in the future. And then follow up!

Meet as many people as you can this first meeting. Try out your introduction, pass out brochures and cards, find out about the group and the purpose of their meetings. Most of all, enjoy yourself!

After you have visited several groups, choose one or two to join. Ask about membership dues, monthly or weekly dues and food costs. If you find (after several meetings) that you aren't getting referrals, try again with a new group.

When you get home, add your new contacts to your email and mailing lists. Follow up with a letter or phone call when appropriate. If you find people you'd like to get to know better, invite them to lunch for a focused networking session.

Some places to network:

- Volunteer opportunities
- Classes
- Art openings
- Concerts
- Trade shows
- Library meetings
- Health food stores
- Your kids' school
- Workshops
- Other therapists
- Doctors office
- Waiting rooms
- Elevators
- Airplanes
- Anywhere you go

M*ailing Lists*

"Don't judge each day by the harvest you reap, but by the seeds you plant." Robert Louis Stevenson

Because they never created a personal mailing list, many of my clients lost out on wonderful opportunities. It is so easy to do and will bring instant rewards when used correctly. You can keep your mailing list on a sheet of paper and hand-write labels, or you can use your computer – but there is no excuse not to have a list!

If you have a computer (and almost everyone I know does), keeping track of the addresses is so convenient: who are current clients, prospective clients, the birthdays, the last visit and who referred them to you. If you are computer savvy, put all your accounting into QuickBooks© or ACT© If you aren't computer savvy, just use a word processing program to keep track. Even Microsoft Word© or Microsoft Outlook© has an address book

Sharon, an astrologer, called me for a telephone consulting session. We chatted for a few minutes and I learned she had been in business more than thirty years and was well known in her field. She had moved several times and had to continuously build up a new client base. She wanted to know if I was able to help her market herself after this latest move. I asked how she had let her previous clients know about her move. She hadn't bothered, she told me, so I asked if she had kept track of all her clients using a mailing list. She hadn't.

When I asked about her clients' files, and if she had the addresses, she replied. "Oh, I have everyone's birth information. I've kept 30 years of files, and in case any of my clients ever call again I'll have the initial reading."

I asked how her clients were supposed to find her after several moves. Was she going to track them down via their birth info? "I'm well-known, I write in several publications and I'm on the Internet. They can find me," she assured me.

Now, this obviously competent astrologer had never mailed out even the most basic information with her new address. No wonder she had to completely start her practice again every time she moved. She had made a presumption that her clients would only want in-person readings, and that they would take the trouble to find her through her published articles, so she never bothered creating a mailing list.

Who can tell what difference one mailing a year might have had on her marketing efforts? These are a few ideas Sharon and I brain stormed during one of our sessions:

- Postcards with a 10% discount for phone readings.

- Moving day promotional offer.

- Promotion for a yearly update sent out a month early.

- Mini birthday readings.

- Readings for newborn babies, marriages, milestone birthdays.

- Special readings such as Valentines Day.

- Monthly readings when the Sun sign changes.

The list could go on and on! Now, this astrologer did do some promotions, but she could only market to the clients that came to see her, and she lost the opportunity to tap into her previous clients.

Experts have said that eighty percent of your business will come from your current client base. You must continue promoting yourself to keep your time filled.

So, how will you use a mailing list? Studies show that almost everyone will read a postcard, and that most people will at least open and read a flier. Other mail that looks like a mass mailing runs the risk of being thrown away without even being opened.

Postcards are quick to design, cheap to mail, and have the largest read rate. Send out postcards at least twice per year. You can expect a few phone calls (perhaps up to three percent of the mailing), and you will stay in the forefront of your clients' minds, reminding prospective clients who you are.

You can send postcards either individually or in a mass mailing, and for a variety of reasons.

- Birthday Wishes

- Your business anniversary

- Invitations to parties or open houses

- Client-only specials

- Health and healing tips

- Announcements

- Spring Fling therapy

You can purchase pre-designed postcards from your office supply store and can print them off your computer or at a copy shop.

Emailing is another way to keep in touch with your clients. Always ask if they would like to receive email from you before adding them to your list. Send email about four times a year with announcements, updates on your clinic and special promotions. You can write a newsletter with ongoing news about your practice, and healthy tips for the reader.

Please make sure that you BCC (blind carbon copy) all the recipients so that the other recipients can't see all the email addresses you send to. You can access BCC under the view menu or when choosing your recipients. Emailing is fast, cheap and easy. Get creative. Keep in touch. Use your mailing list.

E^{vents}

"Hope is not a strategy." General Swartzkoff

There are many types of events that you can use to help build your network. The events can range from classes, workshops and seminars to open houses, trade shows and charity auctions. What is most important is that the event meets your objectives and helps you gain more clients. If you are considering hosting an event or participating in a trade show, ask yourself these questions.

- How excited are you about participating in this event?
- What will be your time commitment to this event?
  - How many clients can you expect?
  - What will be your costs?
  - Is it a good fit? Does this fit your image and style?
  - Will this enhance your reputation and allow you to display your skills?

T*rade Shows*

"A bird doesn't sing because it has an answer, it sings because it has a song." Maya Angelou

Trade shows can be a great way to network and meet new people. Small, industry-focused shows seem to work the best.

Before purchasing a booth ask the following questions:

- How much is a booth?

- What will be your lost revenue from closing your practice during the show?

- How many new clients must you get to pay for the cost of the booth and other expenses?

- Will they provide a table? Chairs? Banner? Tablecloths?

- Will they provide the names and address of all attendees?

- Is there printed material that goes with the show? How will they list you? Are there additional advertising opportunities?

- How will they advertise the show?

- What has been the attendance at previous years?

- How many booths will they sell?

- Do they have references from previous years?

- Can you have exclusive rights to your industry? If not, how many competitors will they allow?

- How will the booth be secured after closing?

- What is the set up/break down policy?

- Will refreshments be available during show hours?

- Can you choose your booth space?

- Can you specify who your neighbors are? Or aren't? (It can be helpful or distracting)

- What is the cancellation policy?

- Are there any additional costs for you or the participants? (Parking, entry fees, adjoining workshops etc.)

Promote yourself three weeks before the show, and mail invitations to everyone you know. Invite them to your booth and have snacks or freebies for your clients. Ask them to bring a friend. Work on creating energy around your booth before the event even starts!

When you work a trade show, go to your booth ready to network and meet new people! Set up your table so that you are standing to the front or to the side of it and can approach people. Don't sit behind your table. It gives the impression you'd rather be elsewhere. Have something that will bring people into your booth like candy or cookies. Put out some fresh flowers, a colorful tablecloth and a banner.

Collect business cards, or at least names and addresses and register people for a free drawing you will hold at the end of the show (need not be present to win). Give away one of your sessions. Put all the names onto your mailing list and follow up with a letter. The letter could include thanks for visiting your booth and a 20% discount for their first session.

Be as alert and cheery at the end of the day as you are at the start. Smile, using all your networking skills. Walk around to the other booths during the slow times, pass out your cards, and talk to people. Network! Consider offering a special promotional discount for other booth owners.

Even if you don't purchase a booth at a trade show, you can still go and do the networking. Use every chance to meet new people and pass out your cards.

And after the show, follow up, follow up, follow up!

*O*pen Houses

"A goal is a dream with a deadline." Napoleon Hill

Open houses are a great way to promote yourself. Think of them as a party for your existing and prospective clients. They give everyone a chance to ask questions and see your office space.

When planning an open house, consider the following:

- Offer refreshments with an assortment of food and drink to encourage people to stay.

- Give a short presentation of your work and explain your services.

- Plan a simple networking exercise so everyone can meet each other.

- Ask a friend to play the guitar or have music in the background.

- Double check that your restrooms are clean with plenty of supplies.

- Collect business cards and do a drawing.

- Offer a discount for anyone who books a session.

You can have focused open houses and invite specific groups. For instance, you could invite all the businesses in your area, all your peers in a related industry, or have a client appreciation evening. Invite practitioners from other locations, specialties or areas of expertise. These practitioners could turn out to be your best referral networks.

Send out postcards four weeks, and again one week, in advance. Send a press release! Ask for RSVP's and have a small gift for anyone who brings a friend. It doesn't have to be expensive; bake cookies, go to the dollar store for ideas, give small soaps or coupons for a free 15-minute session.

Public Speaking

"If you have an important point to make, don't try to be subtle or clever. Use a pile driver. Hit the point once. Then come back and hit it again. Then hit it a third time a tremendous whack." Winston Churchill

Giving a presentation about your work can be the fastest way to build up your practice. You can speak directly to many people at the same time, and offer a question and answer session. What a great opportunity to explain exactly what you do and how it will benefit them. Choose a topic to speak about and spend the next few months developing it. Becoming an expert in your niche.

Many of us are frightened at the prospect of speaking in front of others, so start small and informally. Take a public speaking class if you need some encouragement. Speak to your networking group where you know most of the people. This will help you feel more relaxed as a beginning speaker.

Hold a small class in your office. Give a presentation at your open house.

There are always many clubs and organizations looking for free speakers. Health food stores often have informational evenings, look up the list of the networking clubs and ask if you can speak. Have a brief outline of your talk, do a demonstration and allow questions. Give out your promotional materials with a coupon and remember to collect business cards from others!

When speaking, plant your feet. Keep your arms by your side except for specific gestures. Maintain eye contact with audience members and speak from the heart!

First Impressions

"First impressions are often the truest, as we find (not infrequently) to our cost, when we have been wheedled out of them by plausible professions or studied actions. ..." **William Hazlitt**

So, how do you present yourself in public? When introducing yourself, what do you tell people you do? Are you explaining who you are, and what your passion is? Perhaps you talk with them about the classes you have taken and the new skills you've learned. Does your introduction come across as anxious, unsure or unprofessional? Are you dressed in appropriate clothing? Neat? Clean? Attractive?

A good first impression means everything. You will reflect your own self-image in how you present yourself: your wording, your dress, your posture, your speech. We've all heard the saying, "Act As If." Well now, you must act as if you own the world! You must walk, talk and dress as though you are already a confident, experienced professional, even if you are just starting in this career path. Don't worry, the laws of magnetism will sort out the clients that are most drawn to you and you to them. You must trust that you will offer your clients exactly what they are looking for. Don't hold back. Trust yourself. This will give the best first impression of all.

Office Space

"It is not your customer's job to remember you. It is your obligation and responsibility to make sure they don't have the chance to forget you." Patricia Fripp

Some obvious thoughts: Rest rooms should always be neat and clean with easy access. If your office is in your home, it should be close to the front door, away from distractions such as children, television, radios and outside noise. A radio or CD player is appropriate if you have quiet, flowing music. Have your address visible from the street with appropriate signage. Check the temperature in your office. Make sure chairs are comfortable. Oil squeaky furniture and doors. Have coat hooks or a rack available. Put business cards and information packets out on a table. Have all your office supplies and client files readily accessible. Check your own neatness. Don't overdo the hair spray or perfume, as some people are allergic. Use live plants to dress up a room. Mostly, have it be a comfortable place you would be happy to come to as a client. I once visited a client who had his office in his laundry room. No kidding! His dirty clothes on the floor gave me enough reason to assume why his business wasn't booming!

Take a look around your space with new fresh eyes. How does it look and feel to a first-time client?

Telephone

*"I've suffered from all of the hang-ups known,
And none is as bad as the telephone." Richard Armour*

The telephone is a great tool in your business when used properly. It can also be a headache, a distraction, and downright rude! Use the phone as a tool to help you, but don't let it run your practice for you.

Set a clear time when you will call clients back, say between 8:00 - 10:00 a.m. Be sure your clients know that you will be returning calls then. Be consistent. And don't stay on the phone if you have a client waiting.

Remember to turn off your telephone ringer when seeing clients.

On the telephone give the impression of being busy but helpful and excited to hear from the caller. Often the telephone gives people anxiety, especially if they have never met you and or just want general information. Make the caller feel comfortable immediately.

Always answer on the second or third ring. Answering too soon makes you seem anxious and bored. Answering after the second ring allows the caller to collect thoughts before you pick up the phone. Answer with a short and concise greeting. Don't go on and on. Answering the phone with your name helps the caller to feel at ease immediately, as though they have a friend who can help.

The caller never needs to do or has to do anything. Gina, a naturopath, called me for help converting her telephone inquiries into appointments. She didn't understand why lots of people called for information, but didn't book with her. When we analyzed what she said on the phone, a negative comment emerged. She used to tell people, "Well you will need to make an appointment with me before we can talk about your condition."

To the caller, this sounded as though Gina was put out when a prospective client wanted to ask for information. She was intimidating her callers! Just by re-wording her request she found that her inquiry call to appointment ratio doubled! Now Gina says "I'd love to talk to you about your condition. Let's make an appointment so that we can talk in person. Can you make it in next week?"

Speak from personal experience when talking on the phone. Your caller can relate to your stories or how you have helped others, but remember to keep names confidential.

Telephone Tips:

- Speak clearly, slowly and take a breath between thoughts. Don't rush your conversation. Since you don't have body language to help you interpret the conversation, allow each person time to think and absorb the thoughts and words.

- Stand up when making a call! Your posture will be better, your lungs will be more open, your voice will sound stronger and you will feel more confident. If you are nervous, pace back and forth to release the nervous energy.

- Leave short messages with the purpose of your call, but don't expect to be called back. State a time when you will call again.

- Remember to smile! Yes, you can hear the smile over the phone! Hang a mirror in front of your phone and check yourself as you answer.

- Be decisive and positive. Don't use words like *maybe* or *I'll try.*

- Hang up after the other person hangs up. (Within reason) Be gentle so the phone doesn't bang back into its cradle.

Making Appointments

"The moment that one definitely commits one's self, then Providence moves, too." Goethe

You would think making appointments should be the easiest thing in the world, yet it can often be the most confusing. What should your hours be? How can you offer the convenience of after- hour appointments without hurting your family?

Don't let your clients dictate when you work. Decide your hours and days when you want to work. Try to set up at least one day or evening after regular business hours to see clients, then, set your hours and stick to it!

When you make appointments, set them up back to back. Fill one day with clients before opening another day. Why? This will use your time wisely, leaving other days free for marketing. It will also start creating an energy in your clinic, which other clients will feel. There's nothing worse than going into an empty clinic that feels as though no one ever comes in. It has dead energy. When you have several clients in a day, they can sense, *There's something happening here – I'm glad I am a part of it of it.* When you have a busy clinic, your clients will meet each other in the waiting room and network, exchange stories and generally affirm to each other they are doing the right thing. They will encourage each other along in their journeys toward health. This will affirm that they are making a good choice by coming to see you and help them feel better about their choices.

Try to book appointments at least three days out. Don't be available for a client the next day unless you have a cancellation. Wouldn't you already have your time booked with marketing efforts such as networking?

One way to book an appointment is to say, "I have one opening Thursday morning and another Friday morning. Would either of these work for you?" Or ask, "Is morning or afternoon better for you? I have a Thursday morning or a Monday afternoon." Take control. Give the illusion that you are a successful busy practitioner, even if you aren't quite there yet – You will be!

Have a clear cancellation policy. Don't let the lazy procrastinator take advantage of you. If someone has a true emergency, then waive your cancellation fees, otherwise set a fee and stick to it! Remind your clients of their appointment and call them 24 hours in advance and confirm. People are much less likely to *skip out* on you if they get a confirmation phone call.

One important step, and sometimes the most intimidating for practitioners, is asking the client if they would like to make the next appointment before they leave the office. Once you book the appointment, give them a card with the appointment scheduled. Your client can always cancel, and at least this way you have a confirmed appointment.

Your Clients

"The principle was right there - you couldn't miss it. The more you did for your customers, the more they did for us." Debbi Fields

"The magic formula that successful businesses have discovered is to treat customers like guests and employees like people." Tom Peters

The most powerful marketing strategy anywhere you can apply to your small business is to continuously promote and market to both your current and past customers.

The clients that used to do business with you, but are currently inactive, became clients because you solved a problem or improved their lives in one way or another. Your job is to find out why they stopped booking appointments, and see how you can get them to become one of your customers again. Making telephone calls to these ex-clients brings a personal touch to your marketing approach. Call and ask what is going on with them and how they are doing. Why have they stopped coming to you?

Possible reasons may include moving out of town, no longer need your services, or perhaps they were unhappy with pricing or service. Find out so you can learn adjust. Constantly keep in touch with your clients, offer coupons, specials, thank you notes, so that you stay in their mind. You did all the work to get your client, now keep your client!

Ask your clients questions about what additional services or products (books, oil, lotions, remedies) they might like to purchase from you. What ideas do they have that can help you build your business?

Retention

"A problem is a chance for you to do your best." Duke Ellington

Of course the best retention comes from the client getting good results! However, sometimes it will take four to six visits before your client feels a change, and yet they need to continue coming to you during this time to feel the results! It's a Catch 22!

On the initial visit, talk about realistic expectations. Let your clients know they are making a commitment to their health and will have to book several visits before noticing a change.

Involve them in their own healing, so they feel connected to you and the process. Give them a way to chart their progress. Don't assume they know or feel all the changes. Note in their file symptoms and areas of concern, and review these with them before each visit.

Take an interest in how they are feeling and encourage them to notice any changes – emotional, spiritual, physical – perhaps keeping a journal. Maybe they have lots of changes, but haven't taken the time to notice them.

Ask if are doing different therapies. They may not know what therapies are helping which symptoms.

Providing great customer service is one way to ensure you keep your clients. Go the extra step in everything you do and your clients will stay loyal for years. Customer service means nothing more than showing your clients you care about them. Make them feel comfortable and safe (emotionally and physically) and attend to their needs during a session. When greeting your clients, shake their hand or give them a hug, ask if there are special concerns for the day, offer water to drink, talk about their needs and what has changed since the last visit. Give them a moment to get ready for the session, offer them the restroom, give them a moment to get comfortable. And, although it should go without saying, always give your client privacy to undress. Yes, even if you have seen the client before. Yes, even if you are going to massage your naked client. Yes, even if you have seen the client naked many times. Yes, even if. . . even if. . .Let them undress in private and cover up on the table before you enter the room.

If you have an unhappy customer, know that a client will usually express dissatisfaction at least once to the therapist before going elsewhere. The key is to really hear what your client has to say and act on the information so that you can resolve it.

First, ask questions. Ask with an open heart and be ready to hear whatever is offered to you. Don't take their experience – either positive or negative – personally. After all it is their experience, not yours. If your client is upset don't expect a battle or an argument. There is no reason to be confrontational. If you are being approached with anger, match their energy, but not the emotion. This means take their intensity into your own response, like volume of voice and body language, but stay calm, professional, and concerned. Focus on your listening skills and use your eyes, ears and heart. Repeat back what you have heard so that your client knows you understand their concern. Say "I'm sorry you feel that way." Empathize with their feelings. Understand where they are with their emotions, but don't necessarily accept blame. Then ask what you can do to remedy the situation. Refund their money or schedule another session at no charge if necessary. Remember the golden rule: *Do onto others as you would have them do onto you.*

To minimize dissatisfaction, call the client to follow up after every session, listening carefully.

L ifetime value

> *"A man without ambition is dead. A man with ambition but no love is dead. A man with ambition and love for his blessings here on earth is ever so alive."* **Pearl Bailey**

What is the lifetime value of your client?

Let's say you charge $60.00 per hour for your services, and see a client on average once a month. You expect a client to stay with you for about 18 months before no longer needing your services or moving on. Using these figures, your client will spend $1080.00 on your services. Now assume that this client refers two friends to you in the 18 months. That's another $1080.00 per referral, a total of $2160.00, plus the original $1080.00 Then your client also purchases a gift certificate for another friend for $60.00 and books one double session ($100.00) with you.

If the recipient of the gift certificate buys a package worth $500.00 and then..... ?

How much did the original client bring to you in dollars?

$1080 original client

$2160 two friends

$ 60 third friend

$ 500 third friend

$ 100 discounted double session

Total $3900.00

Can you see how these numbers add up? Take care of your clients. Nurture them, enjoy them, thank them. Once you get them you don't want to lose them.

Become an Expert

"Treat people as if they were what they ought to be, and you help them to become what they are capable of being." Goethe

Commit to learning sales and marketing. Read a few books, learn the process. It will help. You will be a better salesperson. What? Are you still not convinced that you should become a salesperson?

Look at it this way. When you want to go purchase something that you know nothing about, say a washing machine or a new computer, you enter the store and look for someone to answer questions. You want someone who can help explain the difference between brands, someone who can tell you how to get the best price, if there are multi-purchase discounts, and if you can qualify for free delivery. *That* is a salesperson. An expert will help you navigate the buying decisions. This is what you must become, an expert in your field, with yourself as your main product. You will be there for your clients to help them make better and wiser purchasing decisions. Become an expert about your field. Read something every day. At the end of five years you will know as much as the greatest teachers. Practice your gift, and stay committed.

117

*P*roduct Sales

"If you don't sell, it's not the product that's wrong, it's you." *Estee Lauder*

Have you ever thought about selling products to your clients? What else can you sell in your practice? Do you use essential oils? Flower essences? Special bath salts? Is there a particular book you like to promote? If you have a passion for a product or two, purchase these items wholesale and resell them. Research through the Internet or call the manufacturer (usually found on the label), and ask how you can set up a wholesale account.

Here are some things to consider when selling products out of your practice.

States have different sales tax regulations regarding services and products. Research your sales tax collections and reporting requirements.

- Your inventory may sit on the shelf for a few months. How much money do you want tied up in this inventory? Don't purchase more than you can sell or keep stored.

- Be wary and aware of the shelf-life.

- How much time will it take to keep the items on my shelf? Ordering, stocking, pricing etc.

Once you have an item or two in your office, show them off! Put them in a display with a nice big FOR SALE sign close-by. Don't presume your clients will know that they are for sale.

Sharon is an acupuncturist who hand-makes bath salts, soaps and candles. She has had her items on a bookshelf in her office, but she rarely sells. The items were clearly priced for sale; however, they were not readily accessible for clients to feel them, smell them, ask questions about the ingredients. When I came to visit her, we set up a small display case (purchased at a local thrift store and spray painted one afternoon), and laid out all the products right by her front door with a hand painted "Gifts for Sale" sign.

Now when clients come to visit, they can easily pick up the products and ask questions. Sharon has found that she now sells several products a week, and is looking forward to the next holiday season.

Sharon enjoys the making and packaging of her products. For her it is a respite from her busy practice. However, be sure that *you* evaluate your own desires carefully before dedicating so much time to selling a product. Don't become over busy, overwhelmed, and distracted from your main objective.

Remember that selling the items is an adjunct to your practice, and will bring in a little pocket money, but don't expect to make your living off selling products! (Unless you concentrate full time on that aspect of your business!)

Competition

*"**Besides winning, the most fun thing is getting out there and mixing it up with friends; it's the competition." Al Unser, Jr.***

*"**No matter what the competition is, I try to find a goal that day and better that goal." Bonnie Blair***

A word about your competition. Sometimes my clients will get upset when their competition lowers their prices or somehow cuts into their business. I want you to consider who your competition really is. Is it another therapist doing what you do in the same town? What if you look at it another way?

You and the other therapists are all educating the public about the holistic industry. The competition you have is trying to find more clients. About 250 million or more people live in the USA today. How many of them do you see every week? Approximately 30% of the population has tried some form of alternative therapy. Many of these people never try it again. Only about 15% of the people in the USA use alternative therapies on a semi regular basis.

Over 85% of the population do not use any alternative therapies at all. Shouldn't we all band together to educate the public? Competition will only help keep the alternative health industry in people's minds. We need to work together to promote ourselves and be glad in each other's successes. As more people are open to holistic living, we will all find more clients.

Some Final Thoughts

"I went for years not finishing anything. Because, of course, when you finish something you can be judged . . . I had poems which were re-written so many times I suspect it was just a way of avoiding sending them out." Erica Jong

We know that we attract those to us who will teach and guide us on our own path. Often they are mirrors, perfectly reflecting back to us the places where we can heal and bring our own selves into balance. Every person in our lives is there for a reason, to support or teach or mirror us, at exactly the right time. It is always an exchange of energy. As you grow and learn, so will your clients. As you change, the makeup of your clientele will change with you. The perfect clients will find you – right here, right now, right where you are – so that you may mirror something back to them and them to you.

Having a practice can be lonely. Although you talk to people every day, not many are in the same situation, as dedicated as you are to building a business. You need to be in your office making calls, and out marketing yourself. You have to keep the long-term goals in mind so that you don't get discouraged. You are more likely to complete goals when they are written, so write them down now and work toward them each day.

Prevent yourself from getting burned out. Grab hold of your creativity. Nurture your spirituality. Keep it light. Trust. Stick to your protocol. Stay true to yourself and your passions. Develop a support system. Stay focused.

Relax, Have Fun, Enjoy. Life is not a race. Everyone will get there in his or her own time, including you.

The Golden Rules

- The secret to sales is listening – and then responding appropriately.
- The key to staying in business is asking for the cashola!
- The #1 way to increase sales is to find new customers.
- It's a numbers game babe! Not everyone will be a client. You just have to get out and talk to more people.
- Tell 'em what you have to sell – don't assume they know.
- Keep your customers happy! They are worth a lot to you.
- Stay in touch with inactive and present customers.
- Ask who, what, when, where, why and how to gain clarity on a situation.
- Network, network, network! And when you have had enough of that, go meet some more people.
- Become the person you admire. It's contagious and charismatic!
- Remember to have fun. It's your life.